Sirtfood Diet for People on The Go

Delicious Recipes To Help You Activate The Skinny Gene, Lose Weight Faster and Start Feeling Healthier Every Day

Lisa T. Oliver

© Copyright 2021 All rights reserved.

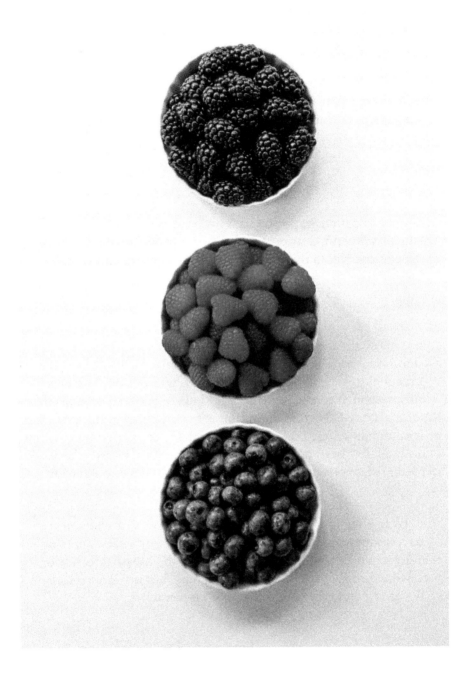

Table Of Contents

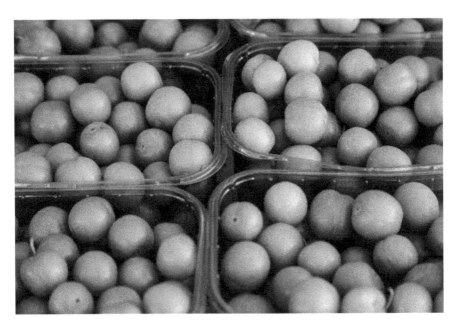

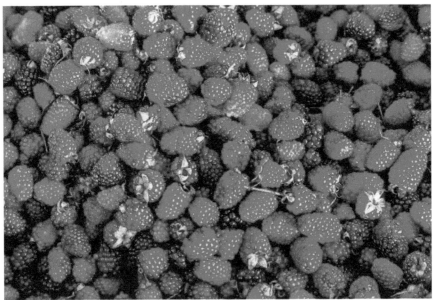

Introduction

The Sirtfood Diet, launched in 2016, has been a trending topic for a while now, with people following the diet very strictly. The creators of the diet suggest that these foods function by activating proteins in the body, referred to as sirtuins. The idea is that sirtuins protect body cells from dying when subjected to stress and regulate metabolism, inflammation, and aging. Sirtuins also boost the body's metabolism and affect its ability to burn fat, providing a weight loss of about seven pounds in a week while retaining muscle. Nonetheless, experts believe that this is solely about fat loss rather than differences in glycogen storage from the liver and skeletal muscle. This diet was developed by UK-based nutritionists, both with MAs in nutritional medicine, and has since gained popularity among athletes and celebrities. Adele and Pippa Middleton are two celebrities who have followed the Sirtfood Diet, and it yielded great results for them. The Sirtfood Diet, like most diets, promotes sustained and significant weight loss, improved health, and better energy. What is it about this diet? Is it just a fad, or is there more to it? Does science back it up? All these questions and more will be answered as you read on. The word "sirt" comes from sirtuins, a group of Silent Information Regulator (SIR) proteins. They boost metabolism, improve muscle efficiency, reduce inflammation, and start the process of fat loss and cell repair. These sirtuins make us healthier, fit, and also help in fighting diseases. Exercise and restrictions on calorie consumption improve sirtuin production in the body.

What Are Sirtfoods?

Sirtuins refer to a protein class that has been proven to regulate the metabolism of fat and glucose. According to research, sirtuins also have a significant impact on aging, inflammation, and cell death.

By consuming foods rich in sirtuins like cocoa, kale, and parsley, you stimulate your skinny gene pathway and lose fat faster.

About the Sirtfood Diet

The Sirtfood Diet plan considers that some foods activate your "skinny gene" and can make you lose about seven pounds in about a week.Certain foods, such as dark chocolate, kale, and wine, contain polyphenols, a natural chemical that imitates exercise and fasting and affects the body. Other sirtfoods include cinnamon, red onions, and turmeric. These trigger the sirtuins' pathway and start weight loss. There is scientific evidence to support this too. The impact of weight loss is higher in the first week. The Sirtfood Diet mainly consists of plant-based foods that are rich in sirtuins to trigger fat loss. The diet is divided into two phases, which can be repeated continuously.The first phase is three days of living on 1000 calories and four days of 1500 calories with lots of green juices.

CHAPTER 1:

Breakfast

1.   Banana Snap

Preparation Time: 3 minutes

Cooking Time: 0 minute Servings: 1

Ingredients:

2.5cm (1 inch) chunk of fresh ginger, peeled

One banana

One large carrot

One apple, cored

½ stick of celery

¼ level teaspoon turmeric powder

Direction:

Place all the ingredients into a blender with just enough water to cover them. Process until smooth

Nutrition:289Calories Total Fat 19gSaturated Fat 2gCholesterol 94mg

Total Carbohydrate 26g Dietary Fiber 4g Protein 8g

2.   Green Egg Scramble

Preparation Time: 3 minutes

Cooking Time: 2 minutes

Servings: 2

Ingredients:

Two eggs whisked

25g (1oz) rocket (arugula) leaves

One teaspoon chives, chopped

One teaspoon fresh basil, chopped

One teaspoon fresh parsley, chopped

One tablespoon olive oil

Directions:

Mix the eggs with the rocket (arugula) and herbs. Heat the oil in a frying pan and pour it into the egg mixture.

 Gently stir until it's lightly scrambled. Season and serve.

Nutrition:

Calories 190 Total Fat 11g Saturated Fat 3.5g Trans Fat 0g

Cholesterol 330mg Total Carbohydrate 7g

Protein 15g

3.   Power Cereals

Preparation Time: 3 minutes

Cooking Time: 0 minute

Servings: 1

Ingredients:

20g buckwheat flakes

10g puffed buckwheat

15g coconut flakes

40g Medjool dates, seeded and chopped

10g cocoa nibs

100g strawberries

100g Greek natural yogurt

Direction:

Mix all ingredients If you are preparing on stock, e.g., for five portions, simply take five times the amount. You can store them for a few days in an airtight tin. If you prefer to eat vegan, use soy yogurt instead of Greek yogurt. Instead of strawberries, you can also use other berries, e.g., raspberries, blueberries, or blackberries.

Nutrition: Calories 130 Total Fat 1g Saturated Fat 0g Total Carbohydrate 28g Protein 6g

4.   Berry Yoghurt

For breakfast as part of your Sirt food diet, we suggest this yogurt, for example:

Preparation Time: 2 minutes

Cooking Time: 0 minute

Servings: 1

Ingredients:

125g mixed berries, e.g., blueberries, strawberries, and blackberries

150g Greek yogurt

25g walnuts, chopped

10g dark chocolate (85%), grated

Directions:

Simply mix all ingredients.

Note: Vegans can also use soy yogurt and vegan chocolate instead of yogurt.

Nutrition:

Calories: 70 kcal

Carbs: 10 g Sugar: 10 g

Fiber: 2 g

Protein: 7 g

5.   Dates & Parma Ham

Preparation Time: 5 minutes

Cooking Time: 3 minutes

Servings: 4

Ingredients:

12 Medjool dates

Two slices of Parma ham, cut into strips

Directions:

Wrap each date with a piece of Parma ham. They are served hot or cold.

Nutrition:

Energy (calories): 845 kcal

Protein: 12.99 g

Fat: 2 g

Carbohydrates: 216.36 g

6.   Braised Celery

Preparation Time: 5 minutes

Cooking Time: 15 minutes

Servings: 4

Ingredients:

250g (9oz) celery, chopped

100mls (3½ fl. oz.) warm vegetable stock (broth)

One red onion, chopped

One clove of garlic, crushed

One tablespoon fresh parsley, chopped

25g (1oz) butter

Sea salt and freshly ground black pepper

Directions:

Place the celery, onion, stock (broth), and garlic into a saucepan and bring it to the boil, reduce the heat and simmer for 10 minutes.

Stir in the parsley and butter and season with salt and pepper. Serve as an accompaniment to roast meat dishes.

Nutrition:

Energy (calories): 225 kcal Protein: 2.24 g Fat: 20.75 g

Carbohydrates: 8.67 g

7.   Cheesy Buckwheat Cakes

Preparation Time: 15 minutes

Cooking Time: 5 minutes Servings: 2

Ingredients:

100g (3½oz) buckwheat, melted and cooled

One large egg

25g (1oz) cheddar cheese, grated (shredded)

25g (1oz) wholemeal breadcrumbs

Two shallots, chopped

Two tablespoons fresh parsley, chopped

One tablespoon olive oil

Directions:

Crack the egg into a bowl, whisk it, and then set aside. In a separate bowl, combine all the buckwheat, cheese, shallots, parsley, and mix well. Pour in the beaten egg to the buckwheat mixture and stir well. Shape the mixture into patties. Scatter the breadcrumbs on a plate and roll the cakes in them. Heat the olive oil in a large frying pan and gently place the cakes in the oil. Cook for 3-4 minutes on either side until slightly golden.

Nutrition:Calories 68 Total Fat 0.6g Saturated Fat 0.1g Trans Fat 0g

Total Carbohydrate 14.4g Protein 1.6g

8.   Red Chicory & Stilton Cheese Boats

Preparation Time: 3 minutes

Cooking Time: 5 minutes

Servings: 4

Ingredients:

200g (7oz) stilton cheese, crumbled

200g (7oz) red chicory leaves (or if unavailable, use yellow)

Two tablespoons fresh parsley, chopped

One tablespoon olive oil

Directions:

Place the red chicory leaves onto a baking sheet.

Drizzle them with olive oil, and then sprinkle the cheese inside the leaves.

Place them under a hot grill (broiler) for around 4 minutes until the cheese has melted. Sprinkle with chopped parsley and serve straight away.

Nutrition:

Calories: 358 calories

9.   Strawberry, Rocket (Arugula) & Feta Salad

Preparation Time: 3 min.

Cooking Time: 0 minutes

Servings: 2

Ingredients:

75g (3oz) fresh rocket (arugula) leaves

75g (3oz) feta cheese, crumbled

100g (3½ oz.) strawberries, halved

Eight walnut halves

Two tablespoons flaxseeds

Directions:

Combine all the ingredients in a bowl, and then scatter them onto two plates.

For an extra Sirt food boost, you can drizzle over some olive oil.

Nutrition:

Calories 680 Saturated Fat 4.5g

Cholesterol 35mg

Total Carbohydrate 41g

Sugars 31g Protein 27g

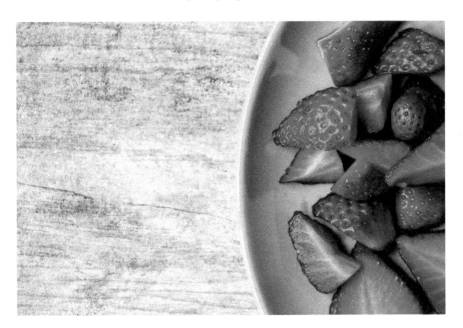

CHAPTER 2:

Lunch

10.   Stir-Fry Asian Shrimp With Buckwheat Noodles

Preparation Time: 10 min.

Cooking Time: 20minutes

Servings: 2

Ingredients:

1/3 pound (150 g) raw jumbo shrimp shelled, deveined

2 Teaspoons of tamari (or soy sauce, unless gluten is avoided)

2 Extra virgin olive oil Teaspoons

3 ounces (75 g) soba (noodles of buckwheat)

Two cloves of garlic, finely chopped

1 Thai chili, finely chopped

One teaspoon of fresh ginger, finely chopped

1/8 cup (20 g) raw, sliced onion

1/2 cup (45 g) of celery with leaves, trimmed and sliced, and leaves set aside

1/2 cup (75 g) chopped green beans

Cup 3/4 (50 g) kale, about chopped

Chicken stock 1/2 cup (100ml)

Directions:

Heat a frying pan over high heat, then cook the shrimp for 2 to 3 minutes in 1 teaspoon tamari and one teaspoon oil. Load the shrimp into a tray. Wipe the pan out with a towel or paper, as you will be using it again.

Cook the noodles for 5 to 8 minutes in boiling water, or as indicated on the box. Drain and pack away.

Meanwhile, in the remaining tamari and oil over medium-high heat, fry the garlic, chili, ginger, red onion, celery (but not the leaves), green beans, and kale 2-3 min. Add the stock and bring to a boil, then cook for a minute or two until cooked but crunchy.

Attach the shrimp, pasta, and leaves of celery to the pan, bring back to a boil, then remove it and serve from fire.

Nutrition:

Energy (calories): 835 kcal

Protein: 75.13 g

Fat: 24.34 g

Carbohydrates: 88.14 g

11.   Miso And Sesame In Ginger And Chili Stir-Fried Greens

Preparation Time: 10 min.

Cooking Time: 20 minutes

Servings: 2

Ingredients:

1 Tablelitre Mirin

Miso paste: 31/2 teaspoons (20 g)

1 x 5-ounce (150 g) Firm tofu block

One celery stalk (40 g), trimmed (about 1/3 cup when sliced)

1/4 cup (40 g) red, sliced onion

One medium (120 g) zucchini (when cut, around 1 cup)

1 Chile Thai

2 Garlic Nails

One teaspoon of fresh ginger, finely chopped

Cup 3/4 (50 g) Kale, Cut

2 Sesame Seed Teaspoons

Buckwheat: 1/4 cup (35 g)

One teaspoon of turmeric powder

2 Extra virgin olive oil Teaspoons

1 Teaspoon tamari (or soy sauce, unless gluten is avoided)

Directions:

Oven gas to 400oF (200oC). Line a small, parchment-paper roasting pan.

Mix both the mirin and the miso. Lengthwise cut the tofu, then diagonally split each slice into triangles in half. Cover the tofu with the miso mix and leave to marinate as the other ingredients are packed.

Slice the angle into the celery, red onion, and zucchini. Chop the chili, garlic, and ginger thinly, and then set aside.Cook the Kale for 5 minutes in a steamer. Discard and set aside.Place the tofu in the roasting pan, sprinkle the tofu with the sesame seeds, and roast in the oven for 15 to 20 minutes until it has been nicely caramelized.Wash the buckwheat in a sieve, and then place it along with the turmeric in a saucepan of boiling water. Cook as directed by package, then drain.Heat the oil in a frying pan; add the celery, onion, zucchini, chili, garlic, ginger, and fry over high heat for 1 to 2 minutes, then reduce to medium heat for 3 to 4 minutes until the vegetables are cooked through, but are still crunchy. If the vegetables start sticking to the pan, you may need to add a tablespoon of water. Add the tamari and kale, and cook for another minute.Serve with the greens and buckwheat when the tofu is ready.

Nutrition: Energy (calories): 384 kcal Protein: 19.03 g Fat: 14.78 g

Carbohydrates: 50.22 g

12. Turkey Escalope With Sage, Capers, And Parsley And Spice Cauliflower "Couscous"

Thin cutlets are ideal, but there are two options to turn it into an escalope if you can just locate turkey breast. You should either use a meat tenderizer, a hammer, or a rolling pin to pound the steak until it's around 1/4 inch (5 mm) thick, depending on how dense the breast is. Or, if you feel that the breast is too thick to work with, and you have a steady hand, cut the breast half horizontally and pound each piece with the tenderizer.

Preparation Time: 10 min.

Cooking Time: 30 minutes

Servings: 2

Ingredients:

Cauliflower: 11/2 cups (150 g), finely chopped

Two cloves of garlic, finely chopped

1/4 cup (40 g) red, finely chopped onion

1 Thai chili, finely chopped

One teaspoon of fresh ginger, finely chopped

2 Spoonful of extra virgin olive oil

2 Tablespoons of turmeric soil

1/2 cup (30 g) of sun-dried, finely chopped tomatoes

1/4 cup (10 g) fresh, chopped parsley

1/3 pound (150 g) steak or turkey cutlet (see above)

Dried sage Teaspoon

1/4 Lemon Juice

Tablet capers

Directions:

Place the raw cauliflower in a food processor to make the "couscous" Pulse to finely chop the cauliflower in 2-second bursts until it resembles couscous. Alternatively, you should use a razor and then finely cut it.

In 1 tablespoon of the butter, fry the garlic, red onion, chili, and ginger until soft but not browned. Attach the cauliflower and turmeric, and simmer for 1 minute. Remove from heat and add the sun-dried tomatoes and half the parsley.

Coat the turkey escalope in the sage and a little oil, and then fry in a frying pan over medium heat for 5 to 6 minutes using remaining oil, turning regularly. Add the lemon juice, remaining parsley, capers, and one tablespoon of water to the pan when cooked through. That will make a cauliflower sauce to serve.

Nutrition:Energy (calories): 1039 kcal Protein: 46.48 g Fat: 69.93 g Carbohydrates: 67.32 g

13.　　Kale And Red Dal Onion With Buckwheat

Preparation Time: 10 min.

Cooking Time: 45 minutes

Servings: 2

Ingredients:

1cup of extra virgin olive oil

1Pound of mustard seeds

1/4 cup (40 g) red, finely chopped onion

Two cloves of garlic, finely chopped

1Teaspoon of fresh ginger, finely chopped

1Thai chili, finely chopped

1Teaspoon of mild curry powder (mean or warm, if you prefer)

2Tablespoons of turmeric soil

11/4 cups of vegetable stock (300ml) or water

1/4 cup (40 g) dried, rinsed lentils

Cup 3/4 (50 g) Kale, Cut

31/2 pounds (50ml) of tinned coconut milk

Buckwheat: 1/3 cup (50 g)

Directions:

Heat the oil over medium heat in a medium saucepan, and add the mustard seeds. When the mustard seeds begin popping, add the onion, garlic, ginger, and chili. Cook until tender, for about 10 minutes.

Connect the turmeric curry powder and one tablespoon, and then simmer the spices for a few minutes. Stir in the stock and bring to a boil.

Add the lentils into the saucepan.

Simmer for another 25 to 30 minutes until the lentils are cooked through and a smooth dal is present.

Add milk to the kale and coconut and simmer for another 5 minutes.

In the meantime, cook the buckwheat with the remaining turmeric tablespoon, as per the box instructions. Drain alongside the dal, and serve.

14.　Aromatic Chicken Breast With Kale And Red Onions And A Chili Salsa Tomato

Preparation Time: 10 min.

Cooking Time: 40 minutes

Servings: 2

Ingredients:

1/4 pound (120 g) of skinless, boneless breast chicken

2 Tablespoons of turmeric soil

1/4 Lemon Juice

1litre, extra virgin olive oil

Cup 3/4 (50 g) Kale, Cut

1/8 cup (20 g) raw, sliced onion

1Teaspoon of fresh chopped ginger

Buckwheat: 1/3 cup (50 g)

TO THE SALSA

1Medium sized tomato (130 g)

1Thai chili, finely chopped

1Mezzanine capers, finely chopped

2 Table cubits (5 g) of parsley, finely chopped

1/4 Lemon Juice

Directions:

Remove the tomato's eye to make the salsa, slice it very well, and preserve as much of the liquid as possible. Mix with chili, capers, lemon juice, and parsley. You could bring it all in a blender, but the end product is a little different.

Heat the oven to 220 ° C (425oF). In 1 teaspoon of turmeric, lemon juice, and a little oil, marinates the chicken breast. Leave on for five to ten minutes.

Heat an oven-proof frying pan until hot, then add the marinated chicken and cook on each side for about a minute or so until pale golden, then move to the oven (set on a baking tray if your pan is not oven-proof) for 8 to 10 minutes or until cooked. Remove from the oven, cover with foil, then leave for 5 minutes to rest before serving.

Meanwhile, boil the kale for 5 minutes in a steamer. Fry the red onions and the ginger in a little oil, then add the cooked kale and fry for another minute until soft but not browned.

Cook the buckwheat with the remaining turmeric teaspoon, as per package instructions. Serve with chicken, vegetables, and salsa.

Nutrition:Energy (calories): 330 kcalProtein: 34.65 gFat: 5.32 g

Carbohydrates: 40.51 g

15.   Harissa Baked Tofu With Cauliflower "Couscous"

Preparation Time: 10 min.

Cooking Time: 60minutes

Servings: 4

Ingredients:

Red bell pepper: 3/8 cup (60 g)

1Half Thai Chili

2 Garlic Nails

About one cubic cup of extra virgin olive oil

Pinch of cumin to the ground

Pinch of coriander

1/4 Lemon Juice

Firm tofu 7 ounces (200 g)

Cauliflower: 13/4 cups (200 g), roughly chopped

1/4 cup (40 g) red, finely chopped onion

A teaspoon of fresh ginger, finely chopped

2 Tablespoons of turmeric soil

1/2 cup (30 g) of sun-dried, finely chopped tomatoes

1/2 cup (20 g) minced parsley

Directions:

Heat the oven to 400oF (200oC).

Slice the red pepper lengthwise around the core to make the harissa, so you have nice flat slices, remove any seeds, then place the chili and one of the garlic cloves in a roasting pan. Add a little oil and the dried cumin and coriander and roast for 15 to 20 minutes in the oven until the peppers are soft but not too brown. (Leave the range on at this setting.) Cold, then mix with the lemon juice into a food processor until smooth.

Lengthwise slice the tofu and then diagonally cut into triangles each half. Place in a small non-stick roasting pan or one lined with parchment paper, cover with harissa, and roast for 20 minutes in the oven — the tofu should have absorbed the marinade and turned dark red.

Place the raw cauliflower in a food processor to make the "couscous" Pulse to finely chop the cauliflower in 2-second bursts until it resembles couscous. Alternatively, you should use a razor and then finely cut it.

Thin out the remaining clove of garlic. In 1 teaspoon of oil, fry the garlic, red onion, and ginger until soft but not browned, then add the turmeric and cauliflower and cook for 1 minute.

Remove from heat and stir in the tomatoes and parsley, which are dried with the sun. Serve with tofu, which is fried.

Nutrition:Energy (calories): 1393 kcalProtein: 46.08 gFat: 112.94 g

Carbohydrates: 65.47 g

CHAPTER 3:

Dinner

16.   Sirtfood Cauliflower Couscous & Turkey Steak

Preparation Time: 10 minutes

Cooking Time: 20 minutes

Servings: 1

Ingredients

150g cauliflower, roughly chopped

garlic clove, finely chopped

40g red onion, finely chopped

1bird's eye chili, finely chopped

1tsp finely chopped fresh ginger

2 tbsp. extra virgin olive oil

2 tsp. ground turmeric

30g sun-dried tomatoes, finely chopped

10g parsley

150g turkey steak

1tsp dried sage

Juice of ½ lemon

1 tbsp. capers

Directions

Disintegrate the cauliflower using a food processor.

Blend in 1-2 pulses until the cauliflower has a breadcrumb-like consistency. In a skillet, fry garlic, chili, ginger, and red onion in 1 tsp. Olive oil for 2-3 minutes.

Throw in the turmeric and cauliflower, and then cook for another 1-2 minutes.

Remove from heat and add the tomatoes and roughly half the parsley.

Garnish the turkey steak with sage and dress with oil. In a skillet, over medium heat, fry the turkey steak for 5 minutes, turning occasionally.

Once the steak is cooked, add lemon juice, capers, and a dash of water. Stir and serve with the couscous.

Nutrition:

Calories 394 Fat: 2 g

Carbohydrates: 12 g Protein: 12 g

Fiber: 0 g

17.   Miso Caramelized Tofu

Preparation Time: 10 minutes

Cooking Time: 35 minutes

Servings: 1

Ingredients

1tbsp mirin

20g miso paste

1* 150g firm tofu

40g celery, trimmed

35g red onion

120g courgette

1bird's eye chili

1garlic clove, finely chopped

1 tsp. finely chopped fresh ginger

50g kale, chopped

2 tsp. sesame seeds

35g buckwheat

1tsp ground turmeric

2 tsp. extra virgin olive oil

1tsp tamari (or soy sauce)

Directions

Pre-heat your over to 200C or gas mark 6.

Cover a tray with baking parchment. Combine the mirin and miso.

Dice the tofu and coat it in the mirin-miso mixture in a resealable plastic bag. Set aside to marinate. Chop the vegetables (except for the kale) at a diagonal angle to produce long slices. Using a steamer, cook the kale for 5 minutes and set aside.

Disperse the tofu across the lined tray and garnish with sesame seeds. Roast for 20 minutes, or until caramelized. Rinse the buckwheat using running water and a sieve.

Add to a pan of boiling water alongside turmeric and cook the buckwheat according to the packet Directions. Heat the oil in a skillet over high heat. Toss in the vegetables, herbs, and spices, and then fry for 2-3 minutes.

Reduce to medium heat and fry for a further 5 minutes or until cooked but still crunchy.

Nutrition:

Calories 273 Fat: 2 g

Carbohydrates: 12 g Protein: 12 g

Fiber: 0 g

18.   King Prawn Stir-Fry & Soba

Preparation Time: 10 minutes

Cooking Time: 25 minutes

Servings: 2

Ingredients:

150g shelled raw king prawns, deveined

2 tsp. tamari

2 tsp. extra virgin olive oil

75 soba

One garlic clove, finely chopped

One bird's eye chili, finely chopped

1 tsp. finely chopped fresh ginger

20g red onions, sliced

40g celery, trimmed and sliced

75g green beans, chopped

50g kale, roughly chopped

100ml chicken stock

Directions:

Warm a skillet over high heat, and then fry for the pawns in 1 tsp. Of the tamari and 1 tsp. Of olive oil.

Transfer the skillet contents to a plate, and then wipe the skillet with a kitchen towel to remove the lingering sauce.

Boil water and cook the soba for 8 minutes, or according to packet directions.

Drain and set aside for later. We are using the remaining 1 tsp. Olive oil, fry the remaining ingredients for 3-4 minutes.

Add the stock and bring to the boil, simmering until the vegetables are tender but still have a bite.

Add the lovage, noodles, and prawn into the skillet, stir, bring back to the boil and then serve.

Nutrition:

Calories 435 kcal

Fat: 2 g

Carbohydrates: 12 g

Protein: 12 g

Fiber: 0 g

19.   Fragrant Asian Hotpot

Preparation Time: 10 minutes

Cooking Time: 15 minutes

Servings: 2

Ingredients:

1 tsp. tomato purée

1-star anise, squashed (or 1/4 tsp. ground anise)

Little bunch (10g) parsley, stalks finely cleaved

Small bunch (1Og) coriander, stalks finely cleaved

Juice of 1/2 lime

500ml chicken stock, new or made with one solid shape

1/2 carrot, stripped and cut into matchsticks

50g broccoli, cut into little florets

50g beansprouts

100 g crude tiger prawns

100 g firm tofu, slashed

50g rice noodles, cooked according to parcel directions

50g cooked water chestnuts, depleted

20g sushi ginger, slashed

1 tbsp. great quality miso glue

Directions:

Spot the tomato purée, star anise, parsley stalks, coriander stalks, lime juice, and chicken stock in an enormous container and bring to a stew for 10 minutes.

Include the carrot, broccoli, prawns, tofu, noodles, and water chestnuts and stew tenderly until the prawns are cooked through.

Expel from the warmth and mix in the sushi ginger and miso glue. Serve sprinkled with the parsley and coriander leaves.

Nutrition:

Calories 434

Fat: 2 g

Carbohydrates: 12 g

Protein: 12 g

Fiber: 0 g

20.   Greek Salad Skewers

Preparation Time: 15 minutes

Cooking Time: 30 minutes

Servings: 2

Ingredients

Two wooden sticks absorbed water for 30 minutes before use

Eight enormous dark olives

Eight cherry tomatoes

1yellow pepper, cut into eight squares

½ red onion cut down the middle and isolated into eight pieces

100g (about 10cm) cucumber, cut into four cuts and divided

100g feta, cut into eight shapes

For the dressing:

1tbsp. additional virgin olive oil

Juice of ½ lemon

1 tsp. balsamic vinegar

½ clove garlic, stripped and squashed

Scarcely any departs basil, finely hacked (or ½ tsp. dried blended herbs to supplant basil and oregano) leaves oregano, finely slashed

Liberal flavoring of salt and crisply ground dark pepper

Directions:

Thread each stick with the plate of mixed greens ingredients in the request: olive, tomato, yellow pepper, red onion, cucumber, feta, tomato, and olive, yellow pepper, red onion, cucumber, and feta.

Place all the dressing ingredients in a little bowl and combine them all. Pour over the sticks.

Nutrition:

Calories 364 Fat: 2 g

Carbohydrates: 12 g

Protein: 12 g Fiber: 0

CHAPTER 4:

Mains

21.   Turkey Escalope With Cauliflower Couscous

Preparation Time: 8 minutes.

Cooking Time: 15 minutes

Servings: 1

Ingredients:

150g cauliflower, roughly chopped

One clove of garlic, finely chopped

40g red onions, finely chopped

1 Thai chili, finely chopped

One teaspoon chopped fresh ginger

Two tablespoons of extra virgin olive oil

Two teaspoons turmeric

30g dried tomatoes, finely chopped

10g parsley leaves

150g turkey escalope

One teaspoon dried sage

Juice of a 1/4 lemon

One tablespoon capers

Directions:

Mix the cauliflower in a food processor until the individual pieces are slightly smaller than a rice grain.

Heat the garlic, onions, chili, and ginger in a frying pan with a tablespoon of olive oil until they are slightly glazed. Add turmeric and cauliflower mix well and heat for about 1 minute. Then remove from heat and add half of the parsley and all the tomatoes, and mix well.

Mix the turkey escalope with the oil and sage. Put the rest of the oil in a pan and fry the escalopes on both sides until they are ready. Then add the lemon juice, capers, remaining parsley, and a tablespoon of water and briefly warm it up. Serve with the cauliflower couscous.

Nutrition:

Calories: 103 Fat: 4g.

Carbs: 26g. Protein: 38g.

22.   Chicken With Kale, Red Onions, And Chili Salsa

Preparation Time: 5 minutes.

Cooking Time: 20 minutes

Servings: 1

Ingredients:

For the salsa:

130g tomatoes

1 Thai chili, finely chopped

One tablespoon capers, finely chopped

5 g parsley, finely chopped

Juice of a quarter of a lemon

For the rest:

150g chicken breast

Two teaspoons turmeric

Juice of a quarter of a lemon

One tablespoon of olive oil

50g kale, chopped

20g red onions, sliced

One teaspoon chopped ginger

50g buckwheat

Directions:

It is best to prepare the salsa first: remove the tomato's stalk, chop it finely and mix it well with the other ingredients.

Preheat the oven to 425 °. In the meantime, marinate the chicken breast in some olive oil and a teaspoon of turmeric.

Heat an ovenproof pan on the stove and sauté the marinated chicken for one minute on each side. Then bake in the oven for about 10 minutes, take out and cover with aluminum foil.

In the meantime, briefly steam the kale. In a small saucepan, heat the red onions and ginger with olive oil until they become translucent, then add the kale and heat again.

Prepare buckwheat according to package instructions, serve with meat and vegetables.

Nutrition:

Calories: 384

Fat: 28.00g.

Carbs: 53g.

Protein: 34g.

23.   Tofu With Cauliflower

Preparation Time: 10 minutes.

Cooking Time: 50 minutes

Servings: 1

Ingredients:

60g red pepper, seeded

1 Thai chili, cut in two halves, seeded

Two cloves of garlic

One teaspoon of olive oil

One pinch of cumin

One pinch of coriander

Juice of a 1/4 lemon

200g tofu

200g cauliflower, roughly chopped

40g red onions, finely chopped

One teaspoon finely chopped ginger

Two teaspoons turmeric

30g dried tomatoes, finely chopped

20g parsley, chopped

Directions:

Preheat oven to 400 °. Slice the peppers and put them in an ovenproof dish with chili and garlic. Pour some olive oil over it, add the dried herbs, and put it in the oven until the peppers are soft (about 20 minutes). Let it cool down, put the peppers together with the lemon juice in a blender, and work it into a smooth mass.

Cut the tofu in half and divide the halves into triangles. Place the tofu in a small casserole dish, cover with the paprika mixture, and place in the oven for about 20 minutes.

Chop the cauliflower until the pieces are smaller than a grain of rice.

Then, in a small saucepan, heat the garlic, onions, chili, and ginger with olive oil until they become transparent. Add turmeric and cauliflower, mix well, and heat again. Remove from heat and add parsley and tomatoes. Mix well. Serve with the tofu in the sauce.

Nutrition:

Calories: 197.3

Fat: 9.4 g.

Carbohydrate: 19.3 g

Protein: 13.5 g

CHAPTER 5:

Meat

24.   Savory Chicken With Kale And Ricotta Salad

Preparation Time: 10 min.

Cooking Time: 40 minutes

Servings: 2

Ingredients:

virgin olive oil, 1 tbsp.

One diced red onion

One finely chopped garlic cove

Juice and zest from ½ lemon

Diced chicken meat of your choosing, 300 g

A pinch of salt

A pinch of pepper

For salad

Pumpkin seeds, two tbsps.

Finely chopped kale, 2 cup

Ricotta cheese, ½ cup

Coriander leaves, chopped, ¼ cup

Parsley Leaves, chopped, ¼ cup

Salad dressing

Orange juice 3 tbsp.

One finely minced garlic clove

 virgin olive oil, 3 tbsp.

Raw honey 1 tsp.

Wholegrain mustard ½ tsp.

A pinch of salt

A pinch of pepper

Directions:

Start by cooking chicken. Heat the oil over medium-high heat and add the onions. Let the onions sauté for up to five minutes. Once the onions turn a golden color, add the chicken and garlic if you'd like to finish quickly, stir-fry for up to three minutes at medium-high temperature, or lower the temperature and let it slowly simmer for up to fifteen minutes. The latter option will result in soft chicken, while the medium-heat stir fry will produce crunchy meat dices.

Next, add the lemon juice, pepper, zest, and turmeric during the last four cooking minutes. While your chicken is cooking, prepare the kale. While you can blanch the vegetable in boiling water for up to two minutes, I'd recommend microwaving with ½ cup of water for up to five minutes to preserve nutrients. Remember, kale is edible raw and cooking; it only serves to achieve the desired flavor and consistency. You can microwave the kale for as short as two minutes if all you need is for it to soften up, and the full five minutes if you prefer that fully-cooked taste.

During the last two minutes of chicken cooking, toss in the pumpkin seeds and stir fry. Remove from heat and set aside.

Mix both dishes into a bowl and add ricotta and the remaining fresh herbs. Enjoy!

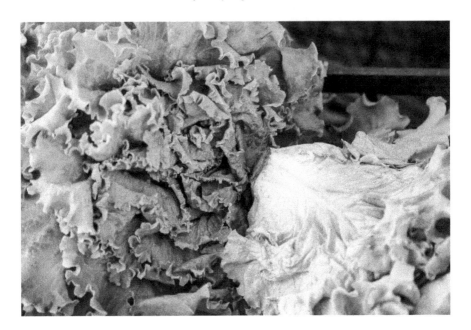

CHAPTER 6:

Sides

25.   Potato Carro Salad

Preparation Time: 15 Minutes

Cooking Time: 10 Minutes

Servings: 6

Ingredients:

Water

Six potatoes, sliced into cubes

Three carrots, sliced into cubes

One tablespoon milk

One tablespoon Dijon mustard

¼ cup mayonnaise

Pepper to taste

Two teaspoons fresh thyme, chopped

One stalk celery, chopped

Two scallions, chopped

One slice turkey bacon, cooked crispy and crumbled

Directions:

Fill your pot with water.

Place it over medium-high heat.

Boil the potatoes and carrots for 10 to 15 minutes or until tender.

Drain and let cool.

In a bowl, mix the milk mustard, mayo, pepper, and thyme.

Stir in the potatoes, carrots, and celery.

Coat evenly with the sauce.

Cover and refrigerate for 4 hours.

Top with the scallions and turkey bacon bits before serving.

Nutrition:

Calories 106 Fat 5.3 g Saturated fat 1 g Carbohydrates 12.6 g Fiber 1.8g Protein 2 g

26.   High Protein Salad

Preparation Time: 5 Minutes

Cooking Time: 5 Minutes

Servings: 4

INGREDIENTS:

Salad:

One 15-oz. can of green kidney beans

2 4 tbsp. capers

3 4 handfuls arugula

4 15-oz can lentils

Dressing:

5 1 tbsp. caper brine

6 1 tbsp. tamari

7 1 tbsp. balsamic vinegar

8 2 tbsp. peanut butter

9 2 tbsp. hot sauce

10 1 tbsp. tahini

Directions:

For the dressing:

In a bowl, stir together all the materials until they come together to form a smooth dressing.

For the salad:

Mix the beans, arugula, capers, and lentils. Top with the dressing and serve.

Nutrition:

Calories: 205 Fat: 2 g Protein: 13 g Carbs: 31 g Fiber: 17g

CHAPTER 7:

Seafood

27.   Baked Fish With Mushroom-Wine Sauce

Preparation Time: 10 minutes

Cooking Time: 10 minutes

Servings: 2

Ingredients:

Cod, haddock, or scrod work equally well in this dish.

Two teaspoons margarine

1 cup chopped mushrooms

Two tablespoons lemon juice

One small garlic clove, minced Dash each salt and pepper

10 ounces fish fillets

1/4 cup each chopped scallions (green onions) and dry vermouth

One tablespoon chopped fresh parsley(optional)

Directions:

Preheat oven to 400°F. In a small skillet, heat margarine until bubbly and hot; add mushrooms, lemon juice, garlic, seasonings, and sauté over high heat, occasionally stirring, until most of the liquid has evaporated.

Place fish in 1-quart casserole and top with mushroom mixture, scallions, and vermouth; bake until fish is opaque and flakes easily when tested with a fork, about 10 minutes. If desired, sprinkle with parsley just before serving.

Nutrition:

Calories: 197 Cal Fat: 4 g

Protein: 26 g Sugar: 2.73 g

28.   Baked Cod Livornese

Preparation Time: 10 minutes

Cooking Time: 30 minutes

Servings: 2

Ingredients:

Two teaspoons olive oil

1/4 cup chopped onion

One garlic clove, minced

1/2 cup chopped mushrooms

1/4 cup white wine

1/2 cup canned Italian tomatoes, chopped

1/4 teaspoon each basil leaves, oregano leaves, and salt Dash pepper

10 ounces cod fillets

Two teaspoons grated Parmesan cheese

One tablespoon chopped fresh parsley

Directions:

Preheat oven to 400°F. In a 10-inch skillet, heat oil; add onion and garlic and sauté until onion is translucent about 1 minute.

Add mushrooms and cook until mushrooms are just tender, about 2 minutes; add the wine and bring to a boil. Add tomatoes and seasonings and cook, occasionally stirring, until sauce thickens, about 2 minutes.

In a shallow 1-quart flameproof casserole, arrange fillets and top with sauce; sprinkle with cheese and bake until fish flakes easily at the touch of a fork, 15 to 20 minutes.

Using slotted pancake turner, carefully remove fish from casserole to serving platter; keep fish warm. Place the soup over medium heat and cook remaining pan juices until reduced and thickened, about 2 minutes; pour over fish and serve sprinkled with parsley.

Nutrition:

Calories: 213 Cal

Fat: 6 g

Protein: 27 g

Sugar: 5.96 g

CHAPTER 8:

Poultry

29.   Chicken In Sweet And Sour Sauce With Corn Salad

Preparation time: 10 minutes

Cooking time: 45 minutes

Servings: 4

Ingredients

2 cups plus two tablespoons of unflavored low-fat yogurt

2 cups of frozen mango chunks

Three tablespoons of honey

¼ cup plus one tablespoon apple cider vinegar

¼ cup sultana

Two tablespoons of olive oil, plus an amount to be brushed

¼ teaspoon of cayenne pepper

Five dried tomatoes (not in oil)

Two small cloves of garlic, finely chopped

Four cobs, peeled

Eight peeled and boned chicken legs, peeled (about 700g)

Halls

6 cups of mixed salad

Two medium carrots, finely sliced

Directions:

For the smoothie: in a blender, mix 2 cups of yogurt, 2 cups of ice, 1 cup of mango, and all the honey until the mixture becomes completely smooth. Divide into four glasses and refrigerate until ready to use. Rinse the blender.

Preheat the grill to medium-high heat. Mix the remaining cup of mango, ¼ cup water, ¼ cup vinegar, sultanas, olive oil, cayenne pepper, tomatoes, and garlic in a microwave bowl. Cover with a transparent film and cook in the microwave until the tomatoes become soft, for about 3 minutes. Leave to cool slightly and pass in a blender. Transfer to a small bowl. Leave two tablespoons aside to garnish, turn the chicken into the remaining mixture.

Place the corn on the grill, cover, and bake, turning it over if necessary, until it is burnt, about 10 minutes. Remove and keep warm.

Brush the grill over medium heat and brush the grills with a little oil. Turn the chicken legs into half the remaining sauce and ½ teaspoon of salt. Place on the grill and cook until the cooking marks appear and the internal temperature reaches 75°C on an instantaneous thermometer, 8 to 10 minutes per side. Bart and sprinkle a few times with the remaining sauce while cooking.

While the chicken is cooking, beat the remaining two tablespoons of yogurt, the two tablespoons of sauce set aside, the remaining spoonful of vinegar, one tablespoon of water, and ¼ teaspoon of salt in a large bowl. Mix the mixed salad with the carrots. Divide chicken, corn, and salad into four serving dishes. Garnish the salad with the dressing set aside. Serve each plate with a mango smoothie.

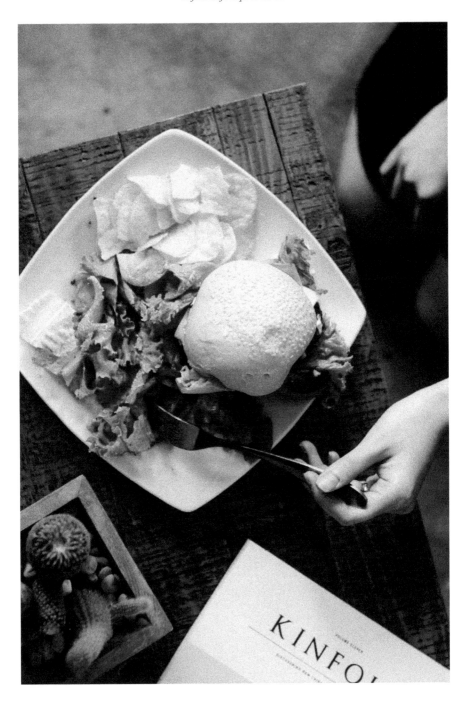

CHAPTER 9:

Vegetable

30.   Classic Pasta Sauce

Preparation Time: 10 min.

Cooking Time: 45 minutes

Servings: 4

Ingredients:

Three onions

Three garlic cloves

Four stems basil

2 tbsp. oil

175 ml wine or vegetable stock

850 g stripped tomatoes (can)

Salt

Pepper

1 tsp. agave syrup

Directions:

Peel and finely slash onions and garlic. Wash the basil and shake dry.

Heat oil during a pot. Braise the onions and garlic during refined warmth for 4–5 minutes. Include the basil and braise quickly.

Add wine or stock and let it come down totally

Chop the canned tomatoes generally with a blade. Put within the pot with tomato fluid and convey it to the bubble. Cook over medium warmth for 25-30 minutes. Expel the basil. Season the sauce with salt, pepper, and agave syrup and use it promptly if vital. Something else, refrigerate and store within the cooler; it remains there for three days.

You'll likewise save the sauce. To undertake to the present, pour the f luid at bubbling temperature into two glasses with a cover (each containing 300 ml) flushed with bubbling water. Close containers promptly and flip around them for five minutes. At that point, stand upstanding and keep calm—the timeframe of realistic usability for around three months.

Nutrition:

Calories90 Total Fat 9g Saturated Fat 3g

Trans Fat 0g Cholesterol 20mg

Sodium 320mg Total Carbohydrate 2g

Dietary Fiber 0g Total Sugars 0.5g

 0g Added Sugars Protein 1g

31.   Shrimp Arugula Salad

Preparation Time: 25 min.

Cooking Time: 0 minute Servings: 4

Ingredients:

10 cups of arugula (baby)

One large-sized avocado (cubed)

Two large lemons (one for juice and therefore the other for wedges)

Five tbsps. of oil or vegetable oil

Half pound large shrimp (cooked)

Salt for taste

Fresh pepper (cracked)

Directions:

Take a bowl and add arugula, avocado, and cooked shrimp. Mix the ingredients and add pepper, two tbsps. of vegetable oil, lemon, and salt consistent with taste. Give the elements a correct mix.Add the remainder of the vegetable oil if you would like to toss the salad again or for coating the arugula.Taste the salad and adjust the seasoning.Serve the salad on a plate by adding wedges of lemon by the side.

Nutrition:507Calories Total Fat 22g Saturated Fat 3g Trans Fat 0g Cholesterol 145mg Sodium 1364mg Total Carbohydrate 57gDietary Fiber 3g Sugars 5g Protein24g

32. Cucumber, Tomato, And Tuna Fish Salad

Preparation Time: 30 min.

Cooking Time: 0 minute

Servings: 2

Ingredients:

Four tbsps. Of peppercorns (fresh, ground)

One and a half cup of tomatoes (cherry variety, add more consistent with your need)

8 oz. of tuna

One small lemon

Salad greens or arugula (any kind that you simply like)

Two medium-sized cucumbers

Directions:

Remove the stems from the cherry tomatoes and wash them properly under running water. Confirm that they're clean. Clean the tomatoes, then dry them by employing a towel or kitchen towel.

Slice the washed tomatoes into half and keep them aside during a bowl.

Equivalent guidelines will get to be followed for cucumbers also. Wash them under cold running water and make them dry by employing a kitchen towel. Cleaning the veggies is extremely important as they're going to be consumed raw within the salad.

Cut the cucumbers consistent with your preferred size and keep them with the tomatoes.

Mix the tomatoes and cucumber.

The animal oil also will be utilized in this salad alongside the fish.

Add the tuna chunks and blend everything gently so that you are doing not break the fish chunks.

Add juice alongside ground pepper and blend well.

Add salad greens to a plate and top it with tuna fish salad.

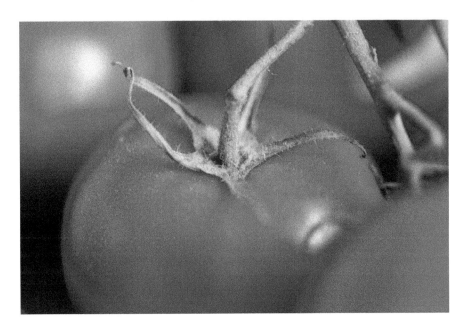

CHAPTER 10:

Soup, Curries and Stews

33.   Medjool Dates Soup

Preparation Time: 10 min.

Cooking Time: 40 minutes

Servings: 1

Ingredients:

7-8 large Medjool dates

½ lb. wolfberries

Two teaspoons honey

1-inch ginger slice

Three glasses of water

Direction:

Peel the ginger slice and set it aside.

Wash the dates and stone' set aside.

Rinse the wolfberries and pat dry. Set aside.

In a saucepan, add water, ginger, dates, and wolfberries. Stir and let it cook for about 40 minutes over a slow flame.

Stir while cooking. Check if the dates are nicely tender. Make sure that water is not dried. If water is reduced too low, then add more water as required.

When done, transfer delicious Medjool date soup into a serving bowl.

Add honey and stir well.

Serve hot.

Enjoy.

Nutrition:

Calories – 543 Fat –0.29 g

Carbs – 146 g Protein – 3.3 g

34.   Chicken And Spring Onion Stew

Preparation Time: 5 min.

Cooking Time: 30 minutes

Servings: 4

Ingredients:

2 lbs. of chicken, boneless, cut into small pieces

0.4 lbs. spring onions, chopped

¼ teaspoon turmeric powder

5-6 medium garlic cloves, minced

1-inch ginger slice, chopped

1cup chicken broth

½ teaspoon freshly ground black pepper

½ teaspoon kosher salt

5-6 tablespoons olive oil

Two teaspoons soy sauce

½ cup red wine

Directions:

Cut the chicken into small pieces. Set aside.

Chop the spring onions into small pieces. Set aside.

Chop the ginger and set aside.

Mince the garlic and set it aside.

Heat olive oil in a large saucepan. Add garlic and sauté until fragrant. Add ginger and stir-fry for few seconds.

Add chicken and salt. Stir-fry until chicken is no longer pink. Cook chicken for 1-2 minutes.

Add black pepper, soy sauce, and turmeric powder. Stir well.

Add spring onion, red wine, and chicken broth. Stir the mixture and cover the pan with a lid. Let the stew simmer over a medium flame for about 10-12 minutes or until the chicken is nicely cooked.

Season soup with black pepper. Mix thoroughly.

Transfer chicken stew to serving dish.

Garnish with the desired ingredient.

Serve hot and enjoy.

Nutrition:

Calories – 2173 Fat – 119 g

Carbs – 22 g Protein – 239 g

35.   Turkey And Buckwheat Soup

Preparation Time: 5 min.

Cooking Time: 40 minutes

Servings: 4

Ingredients:

1½ lbs. of turkey, boneless, in small pieces

One package of buckwheat noodles

1-2 medium carrots, peeled, sliced

4-5 celery stalks, chopped

One small red onion, chopped

5-6 medium garlic cloves, minced

½ cup chicken broth

½ teaspoon kosher salt

One teaspoon freshly ground black pepper

One teaspoon lime juice

Two teaspoons soy sauce

5-6 tablespoons olive oil

3-4 glasses of water

Directions:

In a saucepan, add 3-4 glasses of water and some salt. Bring to boil. Add 1-2 teaspoons of olive oil. Add noodles when water is boiling. Cook noodles until done. Strain the noodles and rinse with cold water. Let aside so that water is drained well.

Cut the turkey into small pieces. Set aside.

Peel the carrots and cut them into small slices.

Chop the onions. Set aside.

Heat olive oil. In a large saucepan

Add onion and sauté until softened.

Add turkey, garlic, and salt.

Stir-fry until turkey is no longer pink.

Add carrot slices and celery stalks. Stir-fry for 1-2 minutes or 4-5 minutes on medium flame.

Add chicken broth. Stir thoroughly.

Cover the saucepan with a lid and cook chicken on low flame for 15-20 minutes or until chicken broth is reduced to half or quarter and turkey and vegetables are tender.

Season with soy sauce, black pepper, and lime juice.

Add noodles and toss everything till combined. Let the noodles simmer for a few seconds. Transfer turkey and noodle soup into serving bowls.

Garnish the soup with the desired ingredient.

Serve hot and enjoy.

Nutrition:

Calories – 4320

Fat – 393 g Carbs – 11 g

Protein – 171 g

36.   Grilled Salmon With Arugula

Preparation Time: 10 minutes

Cooking Time: 30 minutes

Servings: 4

Ingredients:

4 (4 ounces) fillets salmon

1/4 cup olive oil

2 tbsp. fish sauce

2 tbsp. lemon juice

2 tbsp. thinly sliced green onion

1 clove garlic, minced & 3/4 tsp. ground ginger

1/2 tsp. crushed red pepper flakes

1/2 tsp. sesame oil

3 cups arugula

1/8 tsp. salt

Directions:

Whisk together olive oil, fish sauce, garlic, ginger, red chili flakes, lemon juice, green onions, sesame oil, and salt. Put fish in a glass dish, and pour marinade over. Cover & refrigerate for 4 hours.

77 | P a g .

Preheat grill. Place salmon on the grill. Grill until fish becomes tender. Turn halfway during cooking. Serve over a bed of arugula.

Nutrition:

Energy (calories): 545 kcal

Protein: 4.1 g

Fat: 56.83 g

Carbohydrates: 8.66 g

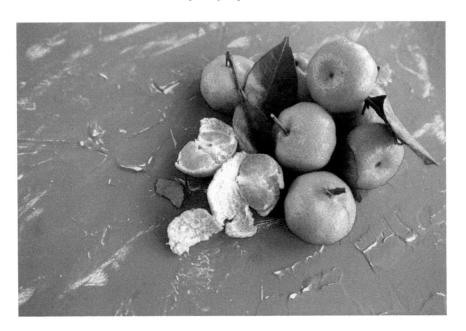

CHAPTER 11:

Snacks & Desserts

37.   Snow-Flakes

Preparation time: 5 minutes

Cooking time: 1 minute

Servings: 2

Ingredients:

Wonton wrappers

Oil for frying

Powdered-sugar

Directions:

Cut wonton wrappers just like you'd do a snowflake.

Heat oil when hot ads won-ton, fry for approximately 30 seconds, then reverse over.

Drain on a paper towel with powdered sugar.

Nutrition:Net carbs 10g Fat 3.69g Fiber 3g Protein 3g

38.   Lemon Ricotta Cookies With Lemon Glaze

Preparation time: 15 minutes

Cooking time: 20 minutes

Servings: 2

Ingredients:

2 1/2 cups all-purpose flour

One teaspoon baking powder

One teaspoon salt

One tablespoon unsalted butter softened

2 cups of sugar

Two capsules

One teaspoon (15-ounce) container whole-milk ricotta cheese Three tablespoons lemon juice

One lemon

Glaze:

11/2 cups powdered sugar

3 tbsps. Lemon juice

1lemon

Directions:

Preheat the oven to 375°F.

In a medium bowl, combine the salt, flour, and baking powder. Set aside.

From the big bowl, blend the butter and the sugar levels. Get an electric mixer, beat the sugar and butter until light and fluffy, about three minutes. Add the eggs one at a time, beating until incorporated.

Insert the ricotta cheese, lemon juice, and lemon zest. Beat to blend. Stir in the dry skin.

Line two baking sheets with parchment paper. Spoon the dough (approximately two tablespoons of each cookie) on the baking sheets. Bake for fifteen minutes, until slightly golden at the borders. Take out from the oven and leave the cookies—remain on the baking sheet for about 20 minutes.

Combine the powdered sugar, lemon juice, and lemon peel in a small bowl and then stir until smooth. Spoon approximately ½ teaspoon on each cookie and use the back of the spoon to disperse lightly. Allow glaze harden for about two hours. Pack the biscuits in a decorative jar.

Nutrition:

Calories 123

Vitamin A and C

Protein 12 g

39.   Homemade Marshmallow Fluff

Preparation time: 1 hour 25 minutes

Cooking time: 10 minutes

Servings: 2

Ingredients:

3/4 cups sugar

1/2 cup light corn syrup

1/4 cup water

⅛ teaspoon salt

Three little egg whites

1/4 teaspoon cream of tartar

One teaspoon 1/2 teaspoon vanilla infusion

Directions:

In a little pan, mix sugar, corn syrup, salt, and water. Attach a candy thermometer into the side of this pan, which makes sure it will not touch the underside of the pan. Set aside.

From the bowl of a stand mixer, combine egg whites and cream of tartar. Begin to whip on medium speed with the whisk attachment.

Meanwhile, turn the burner on top and place the pan with the sugar mix onto heat. Allow combination into a boil and heat to 240 degrees, stirring periodically.

The aim is to find the egg whites whipped to soft peaks and also the sugar heated to 240 degrees at near the same moment. Simply stop stirring the egg whites once they hit soft peaks.

Once the sugar has already reached 240 amounts, turn noodle onto reducing. Insert a little quantity of the famous sugar mix and let it mix. Insert still another small sum of the sugar mix. Carry on adding and mixing slowly, which means you never scramble the egg whites.

After all of the sugar was added to the egg whites, then turn the mixer's rate and keep overcoming concoction for around 79 minutes until the fluff remains glossy and stiff. At roughly the 5-minute mark, add vanilla extract.

Use the lint immediately or store it in an airtight container in the refrigerator.

Nutrition:

Kcal 534 Net carbs 40 g

Fat 35 g Fiber 31 g Protein 22 g

40. Guilt-Free Banana Ice-Cream

Preparation time: 10 minutes

Cooking time: 0 minutes

Servings: 3

Ingredients:

Three quite ripe bananas, peeled and rooted

A couple of chocolate chips

Two tablespoons skim milk

Directions:

Put all the ingredients in a food processor and blend until creamy.

Eat freezes and appreciate afterward.

Nutrition:

Kcal 540 Net carbs 50 g

Fat 45 g Fiber 17 g

Protein 15 g

41.   Perfect Little Snack Balls

Preparation time: 15 minutes

Cooking time: 0 minutes

Servings: 2

Ingredients:

1/2 cup chunky peanut butter

Three tablespoons of flax seeds

Three tablespoons of wheat germ

One tablespoon honey or agave

1/4 cup of powder

Directions:

Blend dry ingredients and adding from honey and peanut butter.

Mix well and roll into chunks and then conclude by moving into wheat germ.

Nutrition:

Kcal 200

Net carbs 30 g

Fat 28 g

Fiber 18 g Protein 11 g

42.   **Dark Chocolate Pretzel Cookies**

Preparation time: 10 minutes

Cooking time: 0 minutes

Servings: 2

Ingredients:

1 cup yogurt

1/2 teaspoon baking soda

1/4 teaspoon salt

1/4 teaspoon cinnamon

Four tablespoons butter softened

1/3 cup brown sugar

One egg

1/2 teaspoon vanilla

1/2 cup dark chocolate chips

1/2 cup pretzels tsp. chopped

Directions:

Preheat oven to 350°F.

In a medium bowl, whisk together the sugar, butter, vanilla, and egg.

In another bowl, stir together the flour, baking soda, and salt.

Stir the bread mixture using all the moist components, along with the chocolate chips and pretzels, until just blended.

Drop a large spoonful of dough on a baking tray without slope.

Bake 15-17 minutes, or until the bottom is crisp.

Allow cooling on a wire rack.

Nutrition:

Kcal 800

Net carbs 23 g

Fat 51 g

Fiber 32 g

Protein 43 g

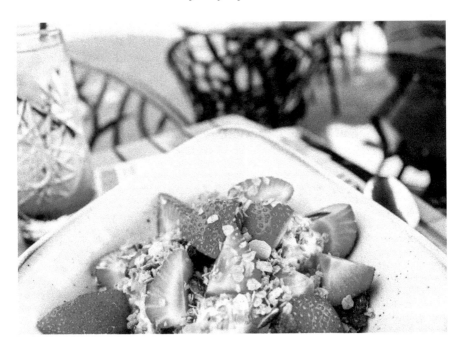

CHAPTER 12:

Desserts

43. Spinach Mix

Preparation time: 10 minutes

Cooking time: 12 minutes

Servings: 4

Ingredients:

1 pound baby spinach

One yellow onion, chopped

One tablespoon olive oil

One tablespoon lemon juice

Two garlic cloves, minced

A pinch of cayenne pepper

¼ teaspoon smoked paprika

Directions:

Heat a pan with the oil over medium-high heat; add the onion and the garlic and sauté for 2 minutes.

Add the spinach, cook over medium heat for 10 minutes, divide between plates and serve as a side dish.

Nutrition:

Calories 20

Sodium 35mg

Carbohydrate 4g

Total Sugars 2g

Protein 1g

44.   Loaded Chocolate Fudge

Preparation time: 10 minutes

Cooking Time: 1+ hours

Servings: 2

Ingredients

1 cup Medjool dates, chopped

Two tablespoons coconut oil, melted

1/2 cup peanut butter

¼ cup of unsweetened cocoa powder

½ cup walnuts

One teaspoon vanilla

Directions

Soak the dates in warm water for 20 – 30 minutes Lightly grease an 8"
square baking pan with coconut oil. Add dates, peanut butter, cocoa
powder, and vanilla to a food processer and blend until smooth. Fold
in walnuts. Pack into the greased baking pan and put in your freezer for
1 hour or until fudge is solid and firm. Cut into 16 or more bite-sized
squares and store in a semi-airtight container in the refrigerator.

Nutrition:320Calories Total Fat 22g Total Carbohydrate 28g Dietary
Fiber 1g Protein3g

45.   Kale Chips

Preparation Time: 5 Minutes

Cooking time: 55 Minutes Servings: 2

Ingredients:

One large head of curly kale, wash, d dry, and pulled from stem 1 tbsp. extra virgin olive oil

Minced parsley

A squeeze of lemon juice

Cayenne pepper (just a pinch)

Dash of soy sauce

Directions:

In a large bowl, rip the kale from the stem into palm-sized pieces. Sprinkle the minced parsley, olive oil, soy sauce, a squeeze of lemon juice, and a tiny pinch of the cayenne powder. Toss with a set of tongs or salad forks, and make sure to coat all of the leaves. If you have a dehydrator, turn it on to 118 F, spread out the kale on a dehydrator sheet, and leave it there for about 2 hours. If you are cooking them, place parchment paper on top of a cookie sheet. Lay the bed of kale and separate it a bit to make sure the kale is evenly toasted. Cook for 10-15 minutes maximum at 250F.

Nutrition:320Calories Total Fat 22g Sodium 50mg Total Carbohydrate 28g Sugars 21g Protein 3g

46.   Moroccan Leeks Snack

Preparation time: 5 minutes

Cooking time: 0 minutes

Servings: 3

Ingredients:

One bunch radish, sliced

3 cups leeks, chopped

1 ½ cups olives, pitted and sliced

Pinch turmeric powder

Two tablespoons essential olive oil

1 cup cilantro, chopped

Directions:

Take a bowl and mix in radishes, leeks, olives, and cilantro.

Mix well.

Season with pepper, oil, turmeric and toss well.

Serve and enjoy!

Nutrition:

140Calories Total Fat 2g Total Carbohydrate 30g

Dietary Fiber 3g Total Sugars 12g Protein 3g

47.　Honey Nuts

Preparation Time: 5 Minutes

Cooking time: 35 Minutes

Servings: 2

Ingredients

150g (5oz) walnuts

150g (5oz) pecan nuts

50g (2oz) softened butter

One tablespoon honey

½ bird's-eye chili, very finely chopped and deseeded

Directions

Preheat the oven to 180C/360F. Combine the butter, honey, and chili in a bowl, then add the nuts and stir them well.

Spread the nuts onto a lined baking sheet and roast them in the oven for 10 minutes, stirring once halfway through. Remove from the oven and allow them to cool before eating.

Nutrition:

140Calories Total Fat 2g

Total Carbohydrate 30g Dietary Fiber 3g

Total Sugars 12g Protein3g

48.   Snack Bites

Preparation Time: 5 Minutes

Cooking time: 35 Minutes

Servings: 2

Ingredients

120g walnuts

30g dark chocolate (85% cocoa)

250g dates

One tablespoon pure cocoa powder

One tablespoon turmeric

One tablespoon of olive oil

Contents of a vanilla pod or some vanilla flavoring

Directions:

Coarsely crumble the chocolate and mix it with the walnuts in a food processor into a fine powder. Then add the other ingredients and stir until you have a uniform dough. If necessary, add 1 to 2 tablespoons of water. Form 15 pieces from the mixture and refrigerate in an airtight tin for at least one hour. The bites will remain in the refrigerator for a week.

Nutrition:Energy (calories): 1830 kcal Protein: 28.63 g Fat: 106.53 g Carbohydrates: 227.26 g

49.   Herb Roasted Chickpeas

Preparation time: 5 minutes

Cooking time: 30 minutes

Servings: 3

Ingredients

One can of chickpeas, drained

1 - 2 tablespoon extra-virgin olive oil

½ teaspoon dried lovage

½ teaspoon dried basil

One teaspoon garlic powder

1/8 teaspoon cayenne powder

¼ teaspoon fine salt

Directions

Preheat oven to 400 degrees F and cover a large baking sheet with parchment paper.

Spread chickpeas out evenly over the pan in a single layer and roast for 30 minutes.

Remove from oven and transfer to a heat-resistant bowl.

Add the olive oil and toss to coat each chickpea. Sprinkle with herbs and toss again to distribute.

Return to oven for an additional 15 minutes.

Let cool for at least 15 minutes before eating.

Nutrition:

Energy (calories): 447 kcal

Protein: 18.56 g

Fat: 16.08g

Carbohydrates: 60.15 g

50. Easy Seed Crackers

Preparation time: 10 minutes

Cooking Time: 60 minutes

Servings: 2

Ingredients:

1 cup boiling water

1/3 cup chia seeds

1/3 cup sesame seeds

1/3 cup pumpkin seeds

1/3 cup Flaxseeds

1/3 cup sunflower seeds

One tablespoon Psyllium powder

1 cup almond flour

One teaspoon salt

¼ cup coconut oil, melted

Directions

Preheat your oven to 300 degrees F.

Line a cookie sheet with parchment paper and keep it on the side.

Add listed ingredients (except coconut oil and water) to the food processor and pulse until ground.

Transfer to a large mixing bowl and pour melted coconut oil and boiling water, mix.

Transfer mix to prepared sheet and spread into a thin layer.

Cut dough into crackers and bake for 60 minutes.

Cool and serve.

Enjoy!

Nutrition:

Energy (calories): 1737 kcal

Protein: 47.27 g

Fat: 154.79 g

Carbohydrates: 64.36

51. Easy And Cheap Quick Cookies

Easiest Chocolate Chip Cookie recipe is a easy chocolate chip cookie recipe that makes super soft chocolate, super yummy chip cookies – no mixer necessary, no chilling needed.

What makes this the easiest chocolate chip cookie recipe?

It uses basic pantry staple ingredients. Also, it is so fast and so easy – no mixer needed no chilling required – that the cookies can be mixed up and baked in less than twenty minutes.

Preparation Time: 10 minutes

Cooking Time: 25 minutes

Servings: 2

Ingredients

2 cups flour rising

Three eggs

1 1/2 cup sugar

200 grams of butter

One milk splash to knead

Two chocolate bars (I use the eagle bars and cut them)

Directions:

Preheat the oven and prepare a plate in butter and then pass it through flour. Mix the flour with the sugar

Add to the flour and sugar, the eggs along with the butter and start mixing.

Incorporate a splash of milk, to be able to shape the dough.

Use all the flour needed to knead

Cut the chocolate and incorporate it into the dough. Then

Once ready, cut into small pieces and crush to shape the cookie. Make it as fine as possible, because it elevates.

Send to the oven 200 degrees only about 5 minutes.

Tip: As with the cake check with a knife to know if it comes out dry. All these came out, it's made them big socks to take less

Bon Appetit!!!

Nutrition:

Calories 56.9

Carbohydrate 29.9

Fat 24.6

Protein 2.4

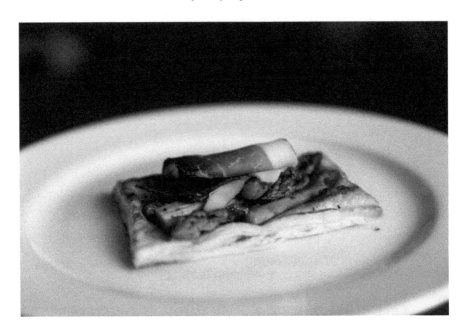

Conclusions

Most diets have been proven to be just a temporary fix. If you want to keep weight off for a good while maintaining muscle mass and ensuring that your body stays healthy, then you need to be following a diet that activates your sirtuin genes: in other words, the Sirtfood Diet.

It is essential to eat a diet that combines whole, healthy, nutritious ingredients with various sirtfoods. These ingredients will all work together to increase the bioavailability of the sirtfoods even further. And there's no need to count calories: just focus on sensible portions and consume a diverse range of foods—including as many sirtfoods as you can and eating until you feel full.

You should also ensure you have a green sirtfood-rich juice every day to get all of those sirtuins- activating ingredients into your body. Also, feel free to indulge in tea, coffee, and the occasional glass of red wine. And most importantly, be adventurous. Now is the time to start leading a happy, healthy, and fat-free life without having to deprive you of delicious and satisfying food.

Lightning Source UK Ltd.
Milton Keynes UK
UKHW020827180321
380564UK00005B/43